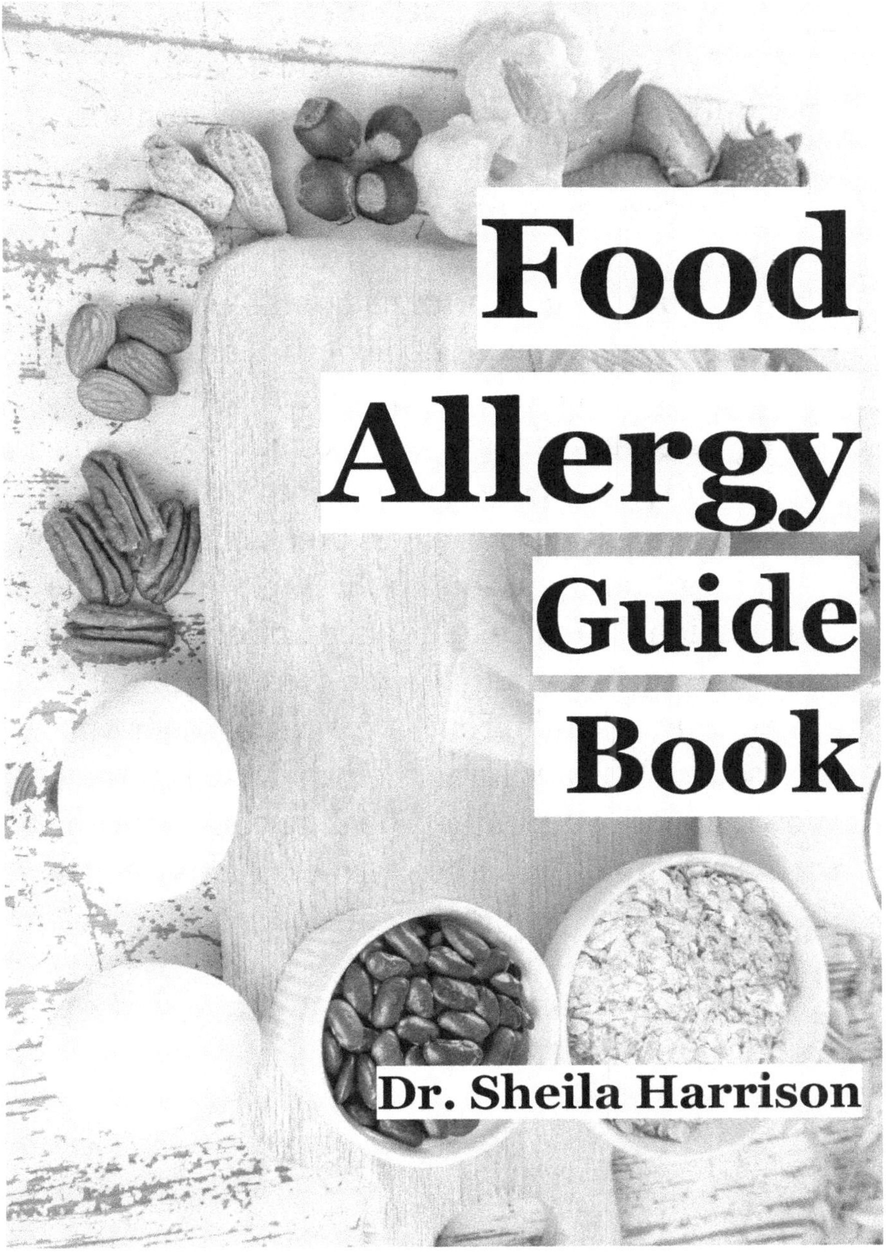

Food Allergy Guide Book

Dr. Sheila Harrison

Disclaimer

This content serves to provide general information about the disease and aims to empower you to seek prompt medical assistance if necessary to prevent complications. It's essential to stress that this information is not a substitute for consulting a qualified physician. The field of medical science is continually evolving, and due to the dynamic nature of medical knowledge, we recommend seeking expert advice if you encounter any inconsistencies or intend to take action based on the information in this content. Never disregard professional medical guidance or delay treatment based on something you've read online, including this material, or from any other online source. Always remember that the internet cannot cure you; rather, healing comes through the guidance of medical professionals and the providence of God.

Table of Content

Overview

Allergies in the U.S. - Statistics & Facts

Allergies arise when an individual is extremely sensitive to an environmental trigger, leading their immune system to mistakenly interpret the trigger as dangerous and consequently overreact to it. The severity of the allergy's symptoms varies, but common ones include a runny nose, watery or itchy eyes, sneezing, a rash, swelling, and difficulty breathing. Typical allergies include latex, pollen, dust, pets and cats, various foods and medications, and insect bites. Approximately 56% of American citizens surveyed recently said that as of 2021, they or a family member were treating or worried about environmental allergies.

According to data collected in 2022, around 61% of American respondents said that they or a household member were managing stress or anxiety. The percentage of American adults in 2022 who reported that they, or a household member, were worried about or receiving treatment for specific health conditions is shown by this data. - Environmental

Section 1
Allergies

Your body reacts to typically harmless things with allergies. The severity of allergy symptoms varies from minor to fatal. Antihistamines, decongestants, nasal steroids, asthma medications, and immunotherapy are among the treatments.

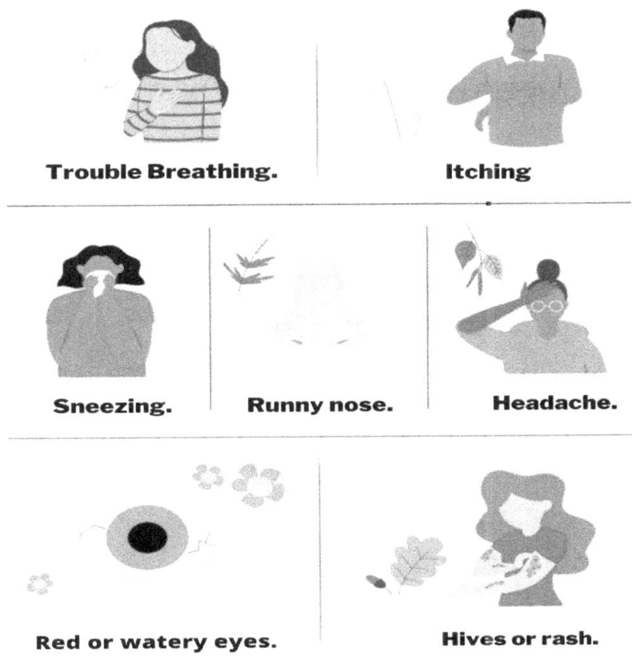

When exposed to some foreign chemicals, allergies cause your immune system to respond.

Your body's response to an unfamiliar protein is an allergy. These proteins, often known as allergens, are typically safe. Your body's defense mechanism, or immune system, overreacts to a protein's presence in your body if you have an allergy to it.

An allergic Reaction

Your body reacts to an allergen by going through an allergic reaction.

When you are allergic, your body produces immunoglobulin E (IgE) in response to the initial exposure to that allergen. Your immune system produces IgE by forming antibodies.

Antibodies containing IgE attach to mast cells, also known as allergy cells, which are found in the skin, respiratory tract, and airways. They also attach to the mucous membrane found in the hollow organs that connect your mouth to your anus (gastrointestinal or GI tract).

The mast cell, also known as an allergy cell, is where the allergens are taken up by the antibodies, who then connect to a specific receptor to aid in their removal from your body. Histamine is released by the allergy cell as a result. Your allergic symptoms are brought on by histamine.

Causes of Allergies

Your immune system's reaction to a foreign material or protein triggers the development of allergies.

Prevalence of Allergies

Having allergies is fairly common. In the US, allergic reactions affect around 55 million people annually. They rank as the sixth most common cause of chronic illness in the US.

Candidates for Allergy

Allergies can affect anyone. You're more likely to have or develop allergies if your biological parents have allergies.

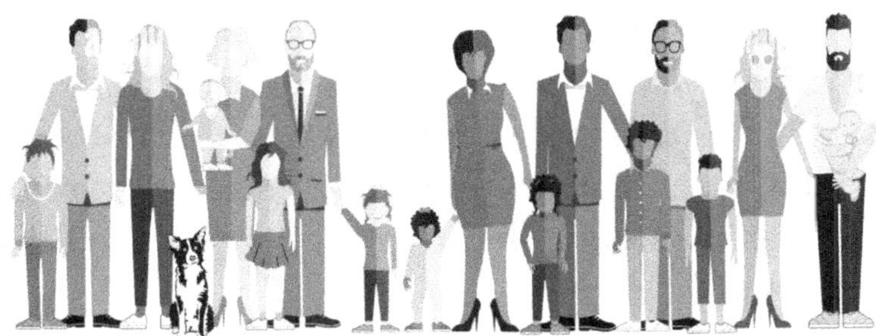

Common Allergy Types, Symptoms and Causes

The most common allergies include:

☑ Some foods

When your body reacts to a particular food, it releases a specific antibody that causes food allergies. Within minutes of consuming the meal, an allergic reaction develops, with potentially serious symptoms. Possible symptoms include:

- ➤ You experience widespread pruritus, or body-wide itching.
- ➤ Localized pruritus refers to itching in just one specific area of the body.
- ➤ Nausea and vomiting.
- ➤ Hives.
- ➤ Swelling in the area around your mouth, encompassing your tongue, neck, or face.

Anaphylaxis is another symptom that you may have if you have an IgE-mediated food allergy. Any one of the aforementioned symptoms or a mix of them may be how it manifests. After consuming a food to which you are allergic, it usually happens within 30 minutes.

The most prevalent food allergies among adults are:

> Milk.

> Eggs.

> Wheat.

> Soys

> Peanuts.

> Tree nuts.

> Shellfish.

> Fish

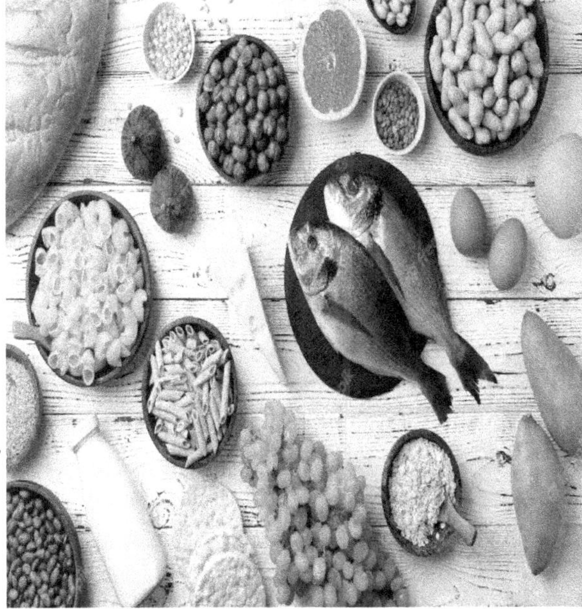

The most typical food allergies in children are:

> Milk.

> Eggs.

> Wheat.

> Soy.

> Peanuts

> Tree nuts.

☑Inhalants

Allergies caused by inhaled chemicals are known as inhalant allergies.

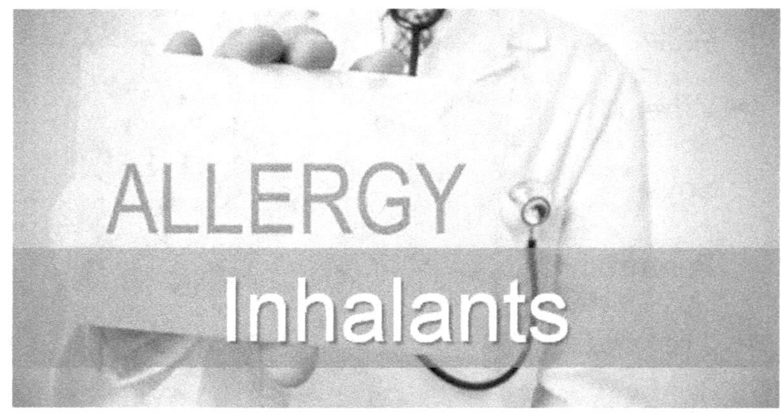

These comprise seasonal allergens as well as perennial allergens, which might affect you all year round.

Symptoms of an inhalant allergy include:

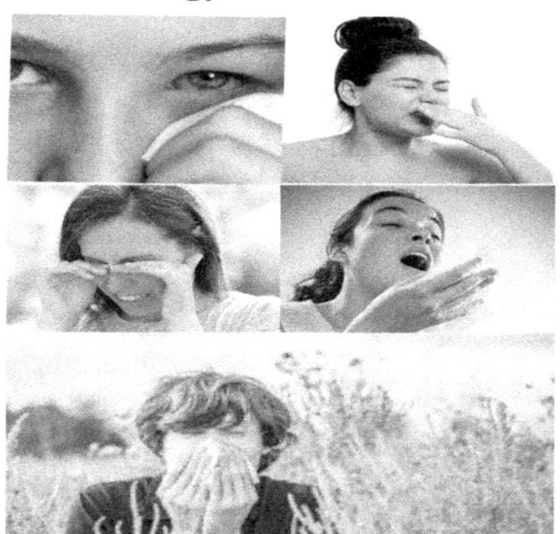

> Runny nose.

> Stuffy nose.

> Itchy nose.

> Sneezing.

> Eyes that itch.

> Teary eyes.

Inhalant allergies have the potential to precipitate or exacerbate wheeze and dyspnea in individuals with asthma.

Among the perennial allergens are:

> Pets: Certain proteins found in animal dander, saliva, urine, and fur can cause allergic reactions in humans..

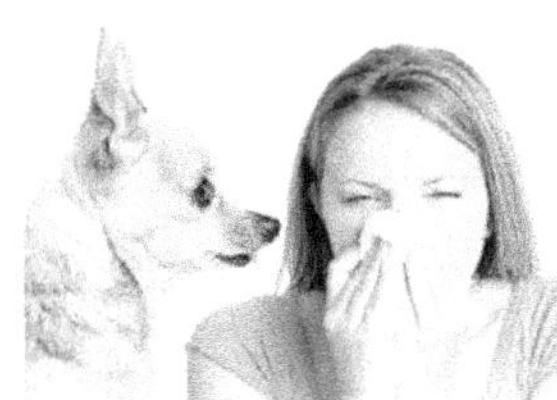

> Dust mites: Spider relatives with eight legs, dust mites are little. Their size is too little for your eyes to see. They are found in the fibers of pillows, mattresses, rugs, and upholstery as well as in dust.

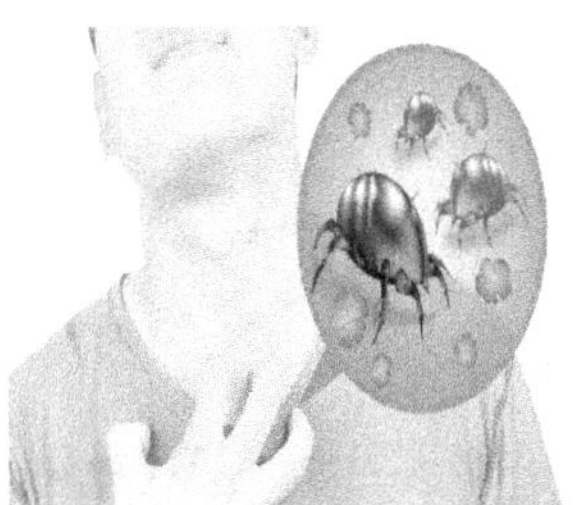

> Cockroaches: 1.5 to 2 inches (in) length, cockroaches are reddish-brown insects. Their saliva, eggs, dead body parts, and excrement all include proteins that can trigger allergic reactions in people.

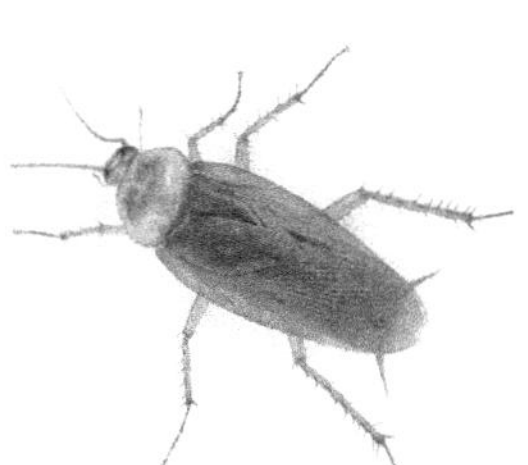

➢ Molds: A mold is a small type of fungus. 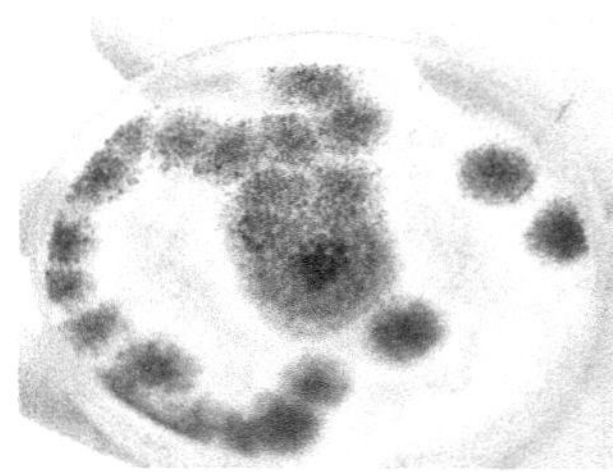 Their spores are airborne and resemble pollen. Aspergillus, Cladosporium, and Alternaria are common mold allergies.

Pollen is one type of seasonal allergy. Pollen is the thin dust-like particles that float in the air or appear on surfaces as tiny grains of grass, trees, or weeds. Pollen from weeds usually appears in the fall, but pollen from trees usually appears in the spring.

☑ Medications

Allergies can occur after taking some drugs. The medications could be prescription, over-the-counter (OTC), or herbal.

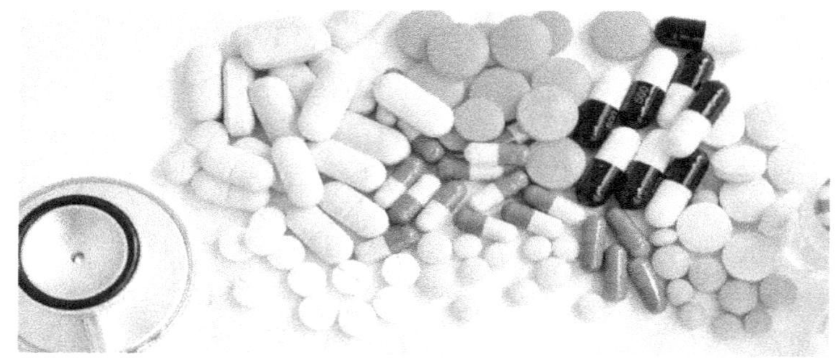

Medications that frequently induce allergies include:

➢ Antibiotics.

➢ Nonsteroidal anti-inflammatory drugs (NSAIDs).

➢ Insulin.

➢ Chemotherapy drugs.

Symptoms include:

➢ Rash.

➢ Hives.

➢ Itching.

➢ Shortness of breath.

➢ Swelling.

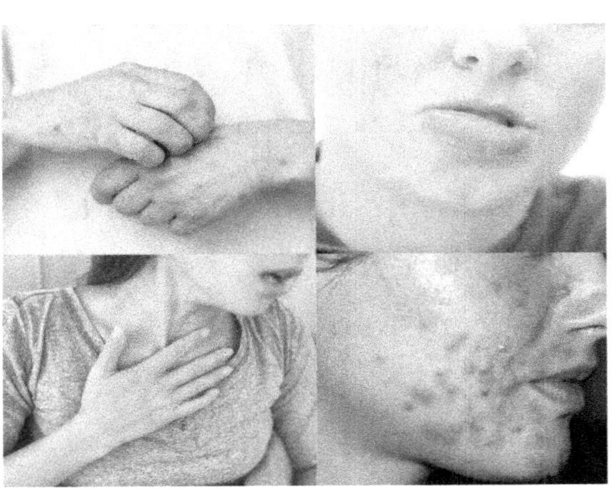

☑ **Latex**

Allergies to natural rubber latex arise from repeated contact.

Typical goods made using natural rubber latex include:

> ➤ Rubber gloves.

> ➤ Balloons.

> ➤ Condoms.

> ➤ Bandages.

> ➤ Rubber balls.

Skin irritation, often known as contact dermatitis, is the most frequent response to latex. It appears as a rash on the skin where the latex came into contact with it. It could appear minutes after coming into contact with latex.

Other symptoms may include:

> ➤ Hives.

> ➤ Runny nose.

> ➤ Itchy nose.

> ➤ Difficulty breathing.

☑ Venoms/stinging insects

Venom is a poison that stinging insects are capable of injecting. An allergic reaction may result from an insect's venom.

The most frequent stinging insects responsible for allergic responses are as follows:

> Bees.

> Fire ants.

> Hornets.

> Wasps.

> Yellow jackets.

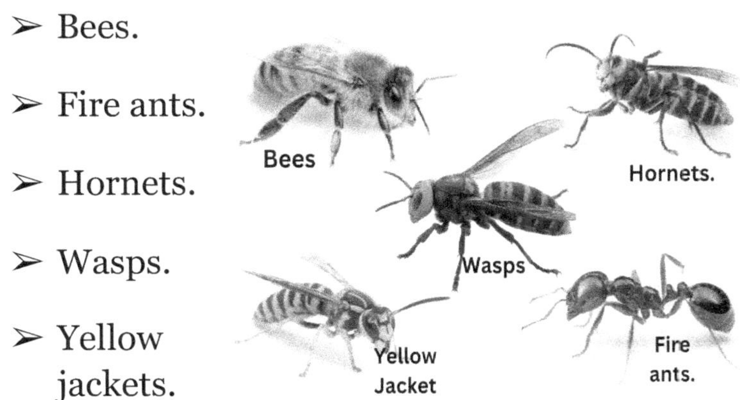

Anaphylaxis is consistent with venom symptoms. They might consist of:

> Trouble breathing.

> Hives.

> Swelling in the mouth, throat, or face.

> Gasping for air.

> Trouble swallowing.

> Quick heartbeat.

> Lightheadedness.

> A decrease in blood pressure.

Can a fever be as a result of allergies?

No, allergies can't cause a fever.

Can One Spread Allergies?

Allergies are not communicable. Your allergies cannot be transferred to another individual.

Now ladies and Gentlemen, because "Food Allergy" is the only topic of interest in this study, buckle up as we delve deeply into the topic.

Section 2

Food Allergies (Subject Matter)

When your body overreacts to the proteins in particular foods or when it responds immunologically to certain foods, food allergies take place. Allergy is the term used to describe this excessive response. Food allergies that are frequently encountered include those to milk, eggs, peanuts, shellfish, fish, soy, tree nuts, and wheat. Avoiding foods that cause the allergy is the best way to treat it. Make an emergency room visit or dial 911 if you experience severe signs of an allergic reaction, such as swelling in your throat.

Types of Food Allergies

Any kind of food can cause an allergy in you.

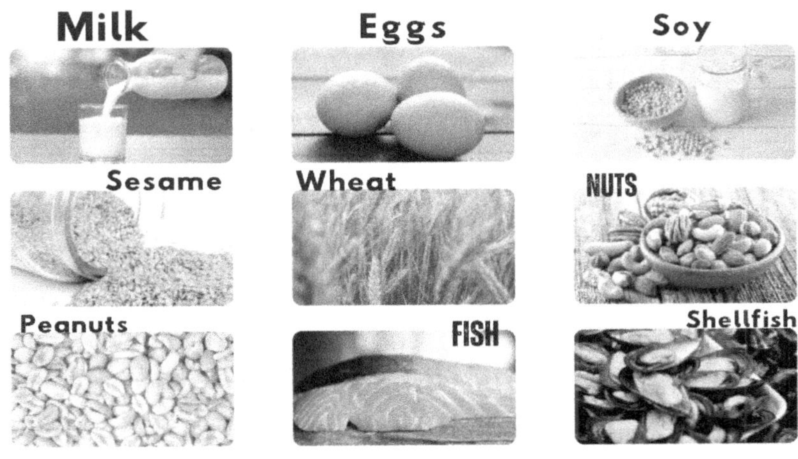

Roughly 90% of all food allergies are caused by Nine different food groups which we will discuss in detail and outline clearly how best to Steer clear of them . These Foods are:

- ☑ Milk.
- ☑ Eggs.
- ☑ Soys.
- ☑ Sesame.
- ☐ Wheat
- ☑ Peanut.
- ☑ Tree Nut.
- ☑ Fish.
- ☑ Shellfish

How prevalent are allergies to certain foods?

Affected Americans number over 50 million with food allergies. Adults who are allergic to food have 4% of them. Up to 6% of kids have a food allergy.

How do my body and food allergies interact?

Dangerous bacteria and viruses are recognized and eliminated by your immune system. When a food allergy occurs, a dietary protein is incorrectly interpreted by the immune system as hazardous. An allergic reaction is brought on by coming into contact with that protein.

Are dietary intolerances and allergies the same thing?

Food intolerances and allergies are two different things. Your immune system reacts to allergens. Having an allergy can be fatal.

Your digestive system responds to food intolerances. If you have an intolerance to a food, you might be able to consume modest amounts of it without developing any symptoms. Although they can be inconvenient, intolerances are typically not harmful.

Symptoms and Causes

Causes of food allergies

Typically, food allergies run in families. You may be more susceptible to a food allergy if you also suffer from other allergic disorders like hay fever or eczema. Moreover, if you have asthma, you are more susceptible to food allergies.

Symptoms of food allergies

Food allergies typically manifest themselves two hours after a meal. Allergies to some foods can cause mild to severe symptoms. When you have an allergic response, you could feel like this:

> ➤ Rash on the skin or hives.
> ➤ Swelling in the eyelids or lips.
> ➤ Tongue swelling, mouth, and throat itch.
> ➤ Difficulties swallowing and a raspy voice.
> ➤ Breathlessness, wheezing, or coughing.
> ➤ Vomiting, diarrhea, and abdominal pain.
> ➤ Losing consciousness or feeling dizzy.

Do food allergies cause any symptoms that are potentially fatal?

Anaphylaxis is the most serious allergic response to a meal. An allergic reaction that progresses quickly and puts your body into shock is called anaphylaxis. Breathing may become challenging or impossible. In the absence of medical intervention, anaphylaxis may be fatal.

Diagnosis and Tests

Diagnosis for Food allergies

When you eat a trigger, food allergies produce comparable symptoms every time. A medical professional might inquire of you in order to diagnose:

- ➢ How long it takes for you to start experiencing symptoms.
- ➢ What you ate, and how much of a certain trigger food.
- ➢ Which symptoms you have and how long they last.

Diagnosing Food Allergies Through Tests

Allergy/immunology physicians can conduct a skin test to confirm a suspected food allergy.

When doing a skin test, your medical professional:

- ➢ Apply a little amount of various allergens (substances that cause allergies) to your back or arms.
- ➢ Creates tiny scrapes or pricks in the allergens.

➢ After the tests have been in place for 15 minutes, measure your response to the allergens.

An allergy is indicated by areas of your skin that become red and itching. To find out what you're allergic to, your healthcare professional uses this information.

RAST stands for radioallergosorbent blood test, which your healthcare professional may also use.

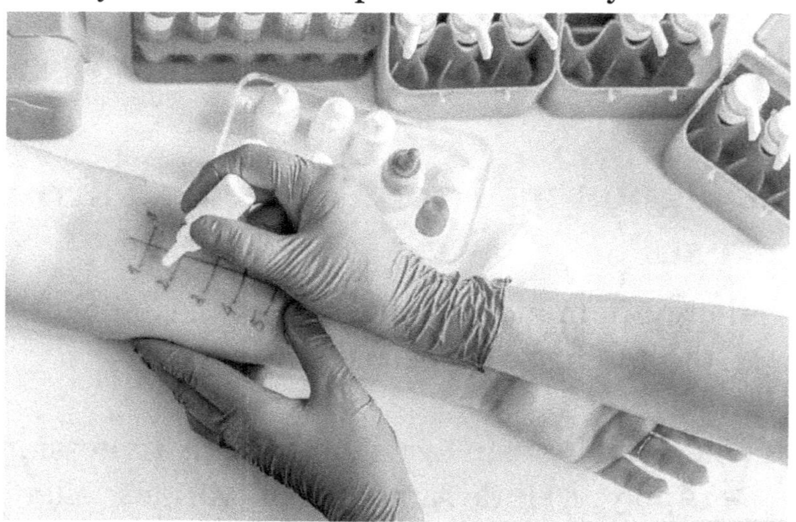

An allergy specific antibody test (RAST) measures the amount of allergen-specific antibodies in your blood. Some antibodies may be elevated in the presence of an allergy.

Management and Treatment

Treatment Options for food allergies

Having emergency drugs on hand, such as epinephrine autoinjectors, in case of an inadvertent intake and reaction, is the best course of action when you are aware of the foods you are allergic to.

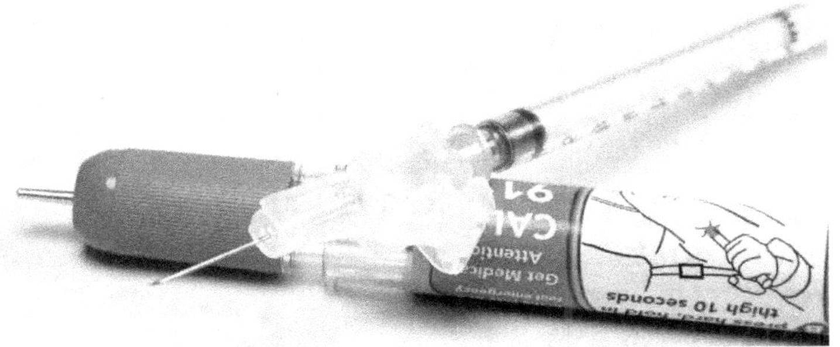

After using an epinephrine auto injector, it's critical to get emergency medical attention right after. It is also advised that you wear a medical alert identification that clearly states your dietary sensitivity.

Medication that lessens the symptoms of your allergic response may be prescribed by your healthcare professional. These medications consist of:

- **Epinephrine** (like EpiPen® or Auvi-Q), a life-saving emergency drug that starts reversing anaphylactic symptoms right away.
- **Antihistamines,** the medications that ease congestion or irritation.
- **Corticosteroids** to reduce swelling if you have a severe allergic reaction.

Avoiding Food Allergy Triggers

You have to closely read ingredient labels on food goods in order to avoid eating the things you are allergic to. All eight of the most prevalent food allergies must be identified on product labels by food makers.

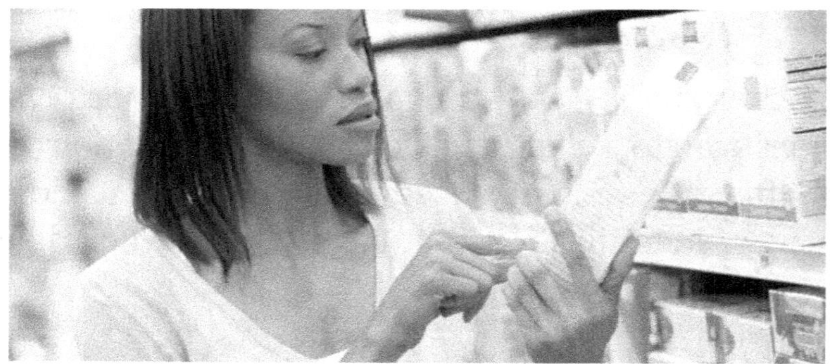

Some labels employ warnings like "made on shared equipment" or "may contain." Speak with your healthcare practitioner if you have any queries about what foods you should and shouldn't be eating.

Food Allergy Prevention

Prevention of Food Allergies

There is no known way to prevent food allergies in adults. In babies, breastfeeding in the first six months of life may prevent milk allergy.

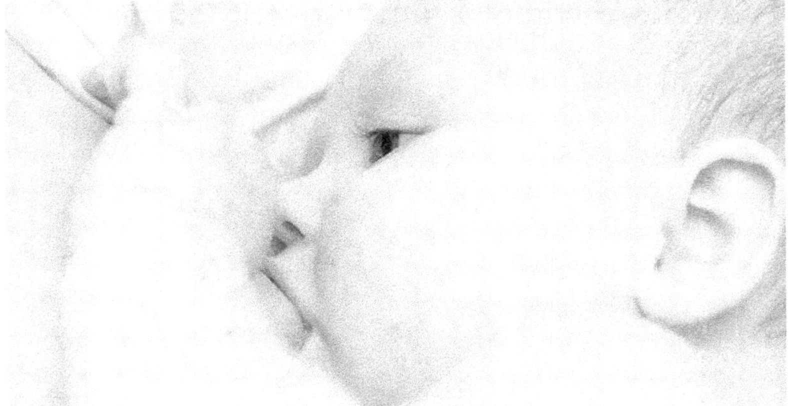

Early introduction of highly allergenic foods such as peanut protein and eggs into the diet may also have a preventative effect. Please discuss with your healthcare provider.

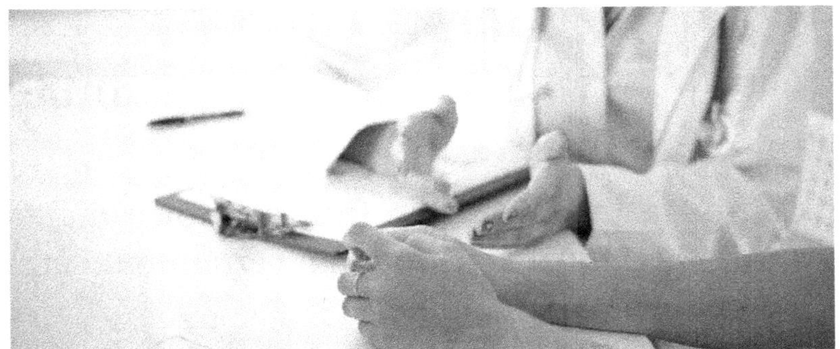

Forecast

How do those who have Food allergies fare in the future?

A food allergy does not have to keep you from being healthy. Avoiding foods and chemicals that trigger allergic reactions is imperative if you have a food allergy.

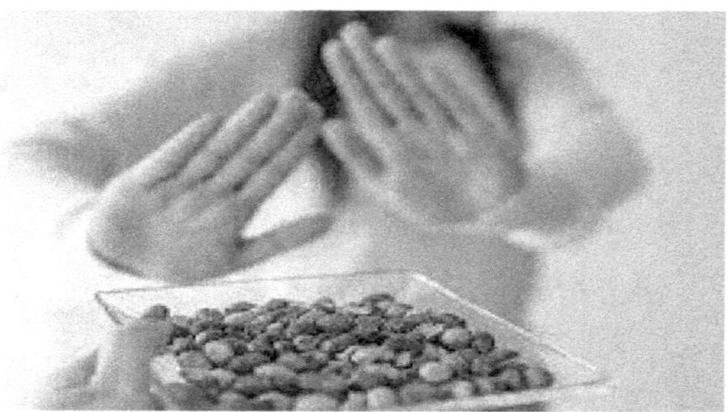

To make up for any nutrients you may have lost by avoiding your trigger foods, you might also need to take a dietary supplement. Prior to beginning a new dietary regimen, see a dietician or your healthcare professional.

When to see Your healthcare provider for a food allergy

Consult a healthcare professional for a diagnosis and treatment if consuming a certain food creates uncomfortable symptoms.

When should I go to the ER

In the absence of medical intervention, allergic reactions may be fatal. Call 911 or visit the ER if you encounter:
> ➤ Breathing problems.
> ➤ Chest constriction.
> ➤ Hives covering your whole body.
> ➤ Lips, hands, or feet tingling.
> ➤ Swelling of the throat that limits breathing.

When your body unintentionally reacts immunologically to particular foods, it might lead to food allergies. An allergic reaction, also known as an immunological response, can result in a number of symptoms such breathing difficulties, swelling, or hives. Anaphylaxis is a potentially fatal reaction that can occur in extreme circumstances. The best approach to manage your allergy is to stay away from the particular foods you've identified as allergens. Pharmacists can recommend drugs to treat allergies and reverse symptoms of anaphylaxis.

Section 3

The 9 Most Common Food Allergies Types.

Allergies can be caused by many foods, although some are more prevalent than others. The proteins (allergens) in nine different foods—milk, soy, eggs, wheat, peanuts, tree nuts, fish, shellfish, and sesame—are linked to about 90% of all severe food allergies.

Since these foods are frequently components in other foods, it takes effort to avoid them, including closely reading labels and taking additional precautions. Even yet, exposures might occasionally occur unintentionally.

Everything you need to know about the most prevalent food allergies is included in this study. It also includes a list of specific items and foods you should stay away from if you have these sensitivities.

Milk Allergy

For newborns and young children, allergies to cow's milk are the most frequent food allergies. Milk allergies are among the most prevalent food allergies in adults, despite the fact that most children eventually outgrow them.One

A small percentage of toddlers under three have a milk allergy (around 2.5 percent).

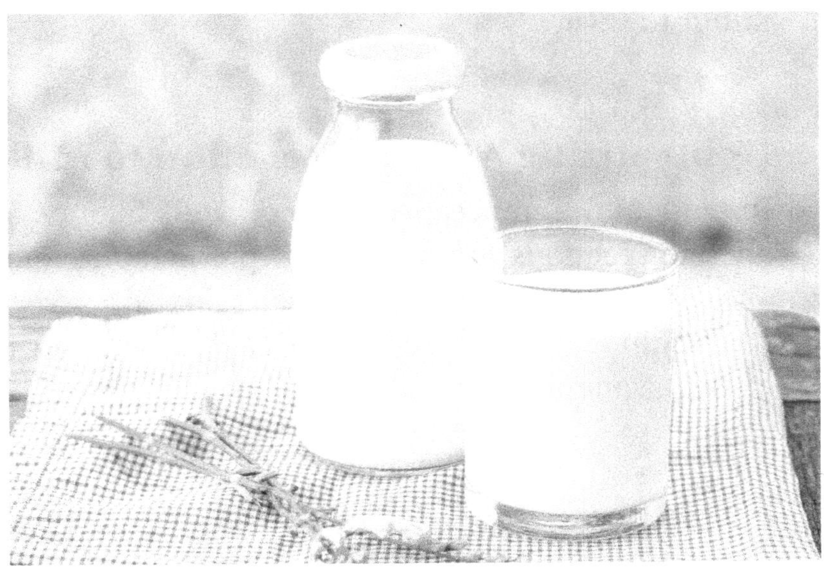

Baked cow milk is tolerated by about 70% of kids who are allergic to cow milk.Two Generally speaking, baked milk is just milk that has been roasted to a high temperature, which breaks down the proteins that cause allergies to cow's milk. It's possible that young children who can consume baked milk

without experiencing an allergic reaction but are allergic to fresh milk will outgrow their milk allergy sooner than those who experience an allergic reaction to baked milk.3

When a person with a milk allergy comes into contact with milk, certain IgE antibodies produced by their immune system attach to proteins in the milk. This sets off the person's immune system, resulting in a range of reaction symptoms from minor to severe.

Neutralizing Allergic Reaction to Milk

Individual differences exist in cow milk allergy, and allergic reactions are not always predictable. A milk allergy reaction's symptoms can vary in severity, from minor symptoms like hives to more serious ones like anaphylaxis.

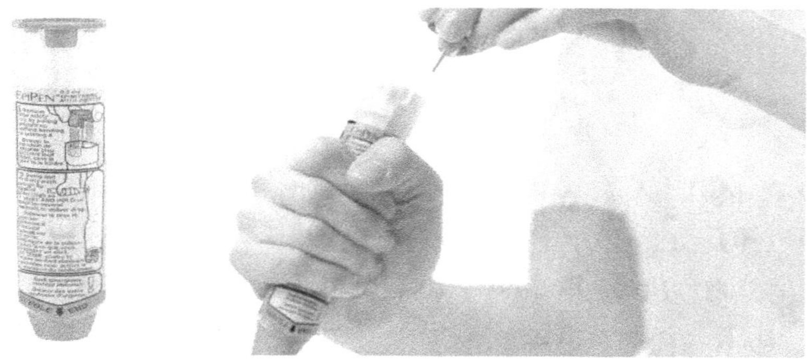

Keep an epinephrine injection kit on you at all times if you have a milk allergy. The primary therapy for anaphylaxis is epinephrine.

Refraining from Eating Foods That Might Include Milk (below are a few)

It's crucial to stay away from cow's milk and food items that contain it if you want to avoid having a reaction. Before consuming anything that you haven't cooked yourself, always check the food labels and inquire about the ingredients.

If you have a cow's milk allergy, your doctor could advise you to stay away from milk from other domesticated animals as well. For instance, the protein in goat's milk is extremely similar to that in cow's milk and can react in those with milk allergies.

According to federal law, packaged foods sold in the United States must indicate all eight major allergens in clear English, either in the ingredient list or in a separate "Contains" statement on the packaging. This includes milk. This makes it simple to determine whether a food item contains milk.

Generally speaking, the ingredients are stated on the package in the order that they appear most frequently in the product. Make sure milk, or a product containing milk, is specified as the third ingredient or later in the list for individuals who avoid baked milk. Whenever in doubt, stay away.

Steer clear of anything with milk or any of the following ingredients:

Cheese	Buttermilk	Casein
Casein hydrolysate	Caseinates (in all forms)	Sour milk solids
Cottage cheese	Cream	Curds
Custard	Ghee	Half-and-half
Tagatose	Yogurt	Lactoferrin
Lactoglobulin	Lactose	Lactulose
Simplesse®	Pudding	Recaldent®
Rennet casein	Milk protein hydrolysate	Whey protein hydrolysate
Lactic acid starter culture	Whey protein hydrolysate	Whey (in all forms)
Sour cream, sour cream solids	Lactalbumin, lactalbumin phosphate	Butter, butter fat, butter oil, butter acid, butter ester(s)
Many restaurants put butter on grilled steaks to	Milk (in all forms including condensed,	Some medications (e.g., psyllium, Advair

add extra flavor. You can't see the butter after it melts.	derivative, dry, evaporated, goat's milk and milk from other animals, low-fat, malted, milkfat, non-fat, powder, protein, skimmed, solids, whole)	diskus, Flovent diskus, some probiotics) contain milk protein.

Other Possible Sources of Milk:

Margarine	Chocolate	Nisin
	Nougat	Sherbert
Artificial butter flavor	Baked goods and desserts	Caramel candies
Tuna fish, as some brands contain casein	Lactic acid starter culture and other bacterial cultures	Snack foods (e.g. chips, crackers, pretzels)
Lactic acid starter culture and other bacterial cultures	Breakfast foods (e.g. cereals, pancakes, waffles)	Non-dairy products, as many contain casein
Pantry Staples (e.g. breads, pasta, tortillas) Shellfish is sometimes	Luncheon meat, hot dogs and sausages, which may use the milk protein casein as	Some specialty beverages (e.g. smoothies, lattes) made with milk substitutes (i.e.,

dipped in milk to reduce the fishy odor. Ask questions when buying shellfish.	a binder. Also, deli meat slicers are often used for both meat and cheese products, leading to cross-contact.	soy-, nut- or rice-based dairy products) are manufactured on equipment shared with milk.

Note: While milk protein can turn up in unexpected places, allergens aren't always present in these foods and goods. Once more, if you're ever unclear about an item's ingredients, read food labels and ask questions.

Will my child's allergy to milk ever go away?

Up to 75% of kids eventually outgrow their milk allergy.5 Children with elevated blood levels of cow's milk antibodies are more likely to continue having the allergy.

Your allergist can assess if a child with a milk allergy is likely to outgrow it with the use of blood tests that evaluate these antibodies.

Over time, consuming baked forms of cow milk may assist promote tolerance or the allergy's remission. Before doing a baked milk challenge at home, be sure to discuss formal challenges with your practitioner.

Egg Allergy

Allergies to hen's eggs are among the most prevalent in infants and early childhood, but they are less common in older kids and adults.

According to experts, up to 2% of kids suffer from egg allergies.

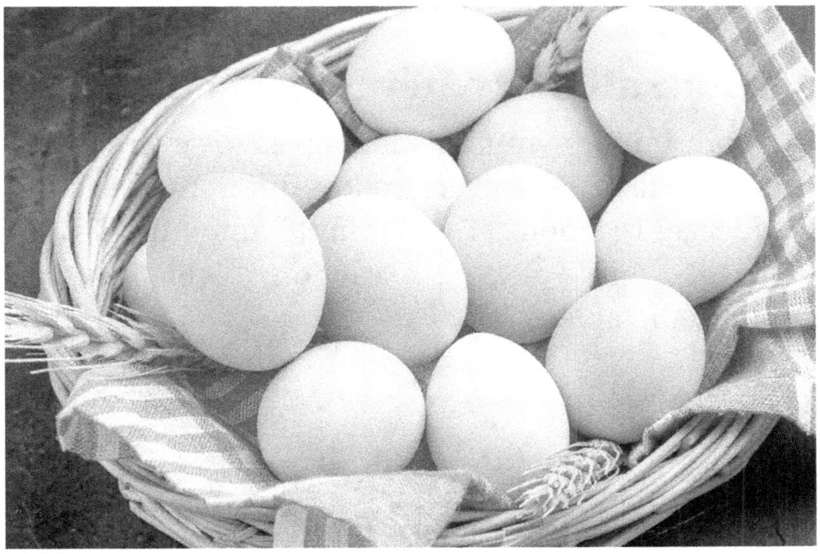

The majority of kids eventually overcome their allergy to eggs (71% by the age of 6), while some people have egg allergies for the rest of their life.

Egg proteins bind to certain IgE antibodies produced by the immune system of an individual who has an egg allergy. This sets off the person's immune system, resulting in a range of reaction symptoms from minor to severe.

A baked egg is tolerated by about 70% of kids with egg allergies.Two The protein that causes egg allergies is disrupted by heating. Over time, tolerance to egg allergy may develop or it may resolve with safe and regular consumption of baked egg products.3 Consult your allergist before attempting baked goods made with eggs at home.

Neutralizing Allergic Reaction to Egg

From minor symptoms like hives to severe ones like anaphylaxis, there are many different types of egg allergic reactions. Even minute amounts of egg can trigger an allergic reaction, which can be unpredictable.

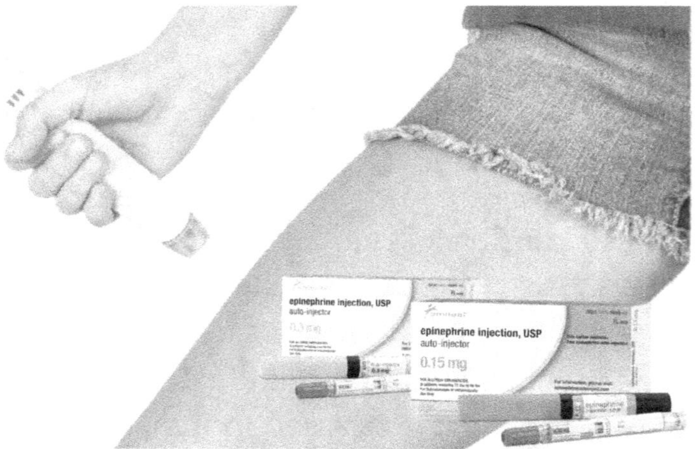

If you are allergic to eggs, carry an epinephrine injection kit at all times. The primary therapy for anaphylaxis is epinephrine.

Refraining from Eating Foods That Might Include Egg (below are some few)

You must stay away from eggs and egg products if you want to stop a reaction. Prior to consuming food that you have not personally cooked, always check the labels and inquire about the ingredients.

Egg allergies are typically caused by certain proteins found in the whites of eggs. You must totally abstain from eating eggs if you have an egg allergy, including the yolk and white. Complete separation of the egg white from the yolk is not possible, even if you are not allergic to the proteins found in egg yolks. The danger of cross-contact never goes away.

If you have an allergy to chicken eggs, your doctor could advise you to stay away from eggs from other domesticated animals as well. A cross-reaction may occur from the eggs laid by ducks, geese, turkeys, and quails.

Listed in plain language in the ingredient list or in a separate "Contains" statement on the packaging, egg is one of the eight major allergens that federal law has to be disclosed on packaged foods sold in the United States. This makes it simple to determine whether a food item contains eggs.

Steer clear of foods that include eggs or any of the following:

Apovitellin	Avidin globulin
Egg (dried, powdered, solids, white, yolk) Eggnog	Albumin (also spelled albumen)
Lysozyme	Mayonnaise
Ovalbumin	Ovomucoid
Ovomucin	Ovovitellin
Surimi	Vitellin
Meringue (meringue powder)	

Eggs are sometimes found in the following:

Chips	Crackers	Hollandaise
Egg substitutes	Nougat	Marzipan
Marshmallows	Lecithin	Ice cream, custard, sorbet
Breakfast foods (e.g. pancakes, waffles)	Breads (may be coated with an egg wash)	Cake decorations or fillings (e.g. buttercream, frosting, mousse)
Baked goods (although some people can	Pretzels (sometimes covered in egg	Souffle Specialty coffee drinks and bar drinks (eggs

tolerate these foods—consult with your allergist)	wash before they are dipped in salt)	can be used in the foam or topping)
Salad dressings	Tortillas	

Pasta: Egg is a component of most cooked pastas produced commercially, including those included in prepared meals like soup. Most dry pastas in boxes don't include eggs. However, some pasta varieties might be prepared using machinery that also handles items containing eggs. Sometimes eggs are not used in fresh pasta. Before consuming any pasta, read the label or inquire about the ingredients.

While egg protein can turn up in unexpected places, allergens aren't always present in these meals and goods. Once more, if you're ever unclear about an item's ingredients, read food labels and ask questions.

Will my child's allergy to eggs ever go away?

Consuming cooked eggs may eventually help the allergy resolve or become more tolerable. Before attempting a formal baked egg challenge at home, make sure to discuss it with your practitioner.

Peanut Allergy

In children under the age of 18, peanut allergy is the most frequent food allergy; in adults, it ranks third. Only 20% of children with peanut allergies eventually outgrow their allergies, which is typically a lifetime condition.

When a person who is allergic to peanuts is exposed to peanuts, certain IgE antibodies produced by their immune system attach to proteins in the peanut. Following oral administration of peanut protein, which activates the immune system, a person may experience mild to severe response symptoms.

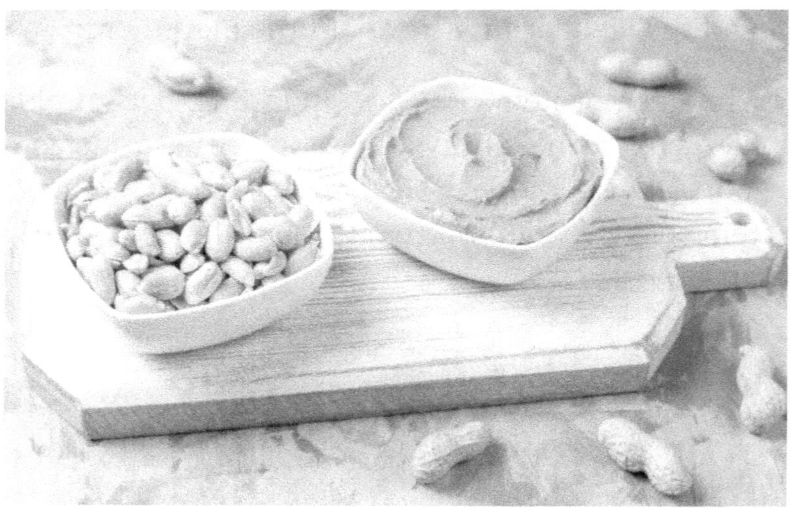

The only food allergy for which a Palforzia medication has been approved by the US Food and Drug Administration is peanut allergy. Although they are not FDA approved, other treatment plans, such peanut oral immunotherapy, are currently being employed to increase a person's tolerance to the peanut protein.

Tree nuts (almonds, cashews, pistachios, walnuts, pecans, and others) are not the same as peanuts. Tree nuts grow on trees. Approximately 40% of children who have allergies to tree nuts also have allergies to peanuts.[2] As members of the legume family of plants, peanuts are grown underground. Beans, peas, lentils, and soybeans are a few other types of legumes. There is no correlation between having a peanut allergy and a higher likelihood of having an allergy to another legume. Nonetheless, individuals with peanut allergy may also have a lupine allergy, which is another legume frequently used in vegan cookery.

Neutralizing Allergic Reaction to Peanut

A severe allergic reaction (anaphylaxis) involving peanuts can be fatal. Even minute exposure to peanuts can result in a severe allergic reaction, as allergic reactions are often unanticipated.

If the afflicted area comes into contact with the eyes, nose, or mouth, it may cause issues and is less likely to result in a severe reaction. Children who are allergic to peanuts may experience an allergic reaction, for instance, if they get peanut butter on their fingers and rub it in their eyes.

If you have a peanut allergy, keep an epinephrine injection device with you at all times. Epinephrine is the first-line treatment for anaphylaxis.

Refraining from Eating Foods That Might Include Peanut (below are a few)

It's crucial that you stay away from peanuts and peanut-derived items if you want to stop a reaction. To determine the ingredients in peanut products, always read food labels.

In the manufacturing and serving processes, peanuts and tree nuts frequently come into contact with one another, which increases the risk of an allergic reaction. Talk about whether you also need to stay away from tree nuts with your allergist.

According to federal law, packaged foods sold in the United States must indicate all eight major allergens in clear English, either in the ingredient list or in a separate "Contains" statement on the packaging. This includes peanuts. This makes it simple to determine whether a food item contains peanuts.

Steer clear of anything with peanuts or any of the following ingredients:

Ground nuts	Beer nuts	Artificial nuts
Mixed nuts	Monkey nuts	Nut pieces
Peanut butter	Peanut flour	Nut meat or nut meal
Peanut protein hydrolysate	Arachis oil (another name for peanut oil)*	Cold-pressed, expelled or extruded peanut oil*
A study showed a strong possibility of cross-reaction between peanuts and this legume, unlike other legumes.	Lupin (or lupine)—which is becoming a common flour substitute in gluten-free food.	Mandelonas (peanuts soaked in almond flavoring)

You don't have to designate highly refined peanut oil as allergenic. Most peanut-allergy sufferers can safely consume this type of peanut oil, according to studies. Seek advice from your physician regarding the avoidance of highly refined peanut oil if you have a peanut allergy.

Avoid cold-pressed, expelling, or extruded peanut oils—also referred to as gourmet peanut oils—if you have a peanut allergy. Small quantities of peanut protein may be present in these less processed oils.

Other Possible Sources of Peanut

Surprisingly, there are peanuts everywhere. Although certain foods and goods may not always contain allergies, it is still advisable to exercise caution.

As you eat something that you have not personally made, don't forget to read the ingredient labels and ask questions. Consume no food if you are unsure of its ingredients.

Even with peanut-free dishes, there is a significant danger of cross-contamination when eating cuisine from African, Asian (particularly Chinese, Indian, Indonesian, Thai, and Vietnamese), and Mexican restaurants.

Some alternative nut butters, such soy nut butter or sunflower seed butter, are made on machinery that also handles peanuts and other tree nuts.

Before consuming these products, get in touch with the maker.

Chili	Egg rolls	Granola
Ice creams	Marzipan	Nougat
Pancakes	Pet food	Trail mix
Enchilada sauce	Glazes and marinades	Specialty pizzas

Grains (such as Muesli cereal)	Sauces such as chili sauce, hot sauce, pesto, gravy, mole sauce and salad dressing	Sunflower seeds (which are often produced on equipment shared with peanuts)
Sweets such as pudding, cookies, baked goods, pies and hot chocolate	Vegetarian food products, especially those advertised as meat substitutes	

Additionally, compost, which is useful as fertilizer for lawns, occasionally contains peanut hulls, or shells. To help you make an informed choice, find out if the contractor you are considering hiring uses peanut hulls in their compost before hiring them.

Will my child's allergy to peanuts ever go away?

Allergy to peanuts appears to be on the rise in children. According to a FARE-funded study, the number of children in the U.S. with peanut allergy more than tripled between 1997 and 2008.[4] Two studies in the United Kingdom and Canada also showed a high prevalence of peanut allergy in school-aged children.

Peanut allergies tend to be lifelong, although studies show that about 20 percent of children with peanut allergy do eventually outgrow their allergy.[1]

Younger siblings of children who are allergic to peanuts may be at higher risk for allergy to peanuts.[5] Your doctor can provide guidance on food allergy testing for siblings. Recent research shows that introducing infants to peanuts early on may help prevent them from developing this food allergy. FARE provides additional resources on this on babyfirst.org.

Soy Allergy

Around 0.4% of newborns in the United States suffer with soy allergy, which is more common in younger children than in older children.One The majority of youngsters eventually overcome their soy allergy, while some people never fully recover from their allergy.

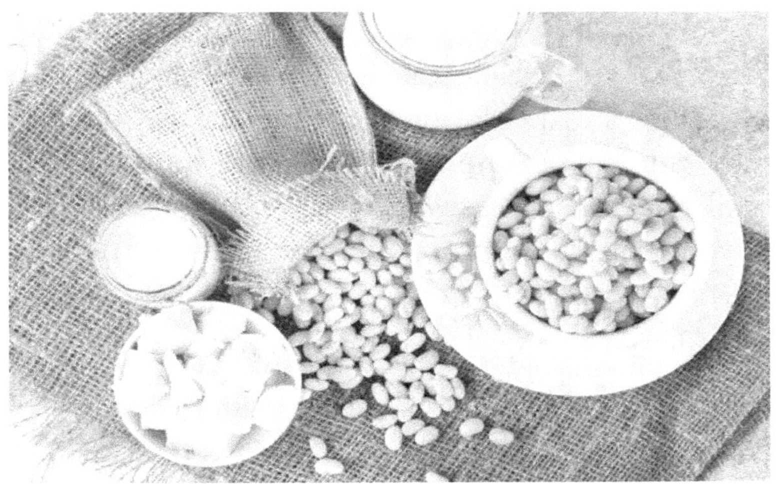

When an individual with a soy allergy comes into contact with soy, certain IgE antibodies produced by their immune system attach to proteins in the soy. This sets off the person's immune system, resulting in a range of reaction symptoms from minor to severe.

The family of legumes includes soybeans. Legumes include peanuts, lentils, beans, and peas. Although people with peanut allergies rarely experience soy reactions, the opposite is not true. Up to 88% of patients with soy allergies either had peanut allergies or were highly sensitive to peanuts, according to one study. When it comes to major allergens like peanuts, tree nuts, eggs, milk, and sesame, those with soy allergies were more likely to be allergic or sensitized to them than to non-peanut legumes like beans, peas, and lentils.

Neutralizing Allergic Reaction to Soy

Although most allergic reactions to soy are mild, they can all be unexpected. Severe and sometimes fatal reactions are possible, albeit they are uncommon (learn more about anaphylaxis).

Carry an epinephrine injection kit at all times if you are allergic to soy. The primary line of treatment for anaphylaxis is epinephrine.

Refraining from Eating Foods That Might Include Soy (below are a few)

You must stay away from soy and soy-derived items if you want to avoid a response. Before consuming anything that you haven't cooked yourself, always check the food labels and inquire about the ingredients.

Although Americans rarely eat soybeans on their own, they frequently employ them in processed foods. A diet that is out of balance may arise from excluding all those foods. Planning for appropriate nutrition can be aided by a nutritionist.

Within the ingredient list or in a separate "Contains" statement on the packaging, packaged foods sold in the United States are required by federal law to declare all eight major allergens in plain language, including soy. This makes it simple to determine whether a food item contains soy. Note: Most soy-allergic patients may tolerate soy lecithin, even though it is not excluded from FALCPA. It is also not usually avoided on a soy-elimination diet.

Steer clear of anything with soy or any of the following ingredients:

Edamame	Miso	Natto
Okara	Shoyu	Soya
Soy sauce	Tamari	Tempeh
Soybean (curd, granules)	Textured vegetable protein (TVP)	Tofu
Cold-pressed, expelled or extruded soy oil*	Soy protein (concentrate, hydrolyzed, isolate)	Soy (soy albumin, soy cheese, soy fiber, soy flour, soy grits, soy ice cream, soy milk,

		soy nuts, soy sprouts, soy yogurt)

An allergen label is not necessary for highly refined soy oil. Studies indicate that most soy-allergic individuals can safely consume soy lecithin and highly refined soy oil. Check with your physician if you must avoid soy lecithin or oil if you have a soy allergy.

Cold-pressed, expedited, or extruded soy oils—also referred to as gourmet soy oils—should be avoided by anyone who is allergic to soybeans. Small amounts of soy protein may be present in some minimally refined products.

A growing number of vegan and vegetarian options, in line with the trend toward plant-based diets, use soy as a meat substitute to give their goods an equivalent feel. Verify the label at all times!

The following items occasionally include soy:

Vegetable gum	Vegetable starch	Vegetable broth
Asian cuisine (including Chinese, Indian, Indonesian, Thai and Vietnamese)—even if you order a	Grains prepared with soy (e.g. cereals, breads, chips, crackers, pasta, rice, tortillas and rice)	

| soy-free item, there is high risk of cross-contact | | |

Some unexpected sources of soybeans and soy products

Baked goods	Cereals	Cookies
Crackers	Pet food	Sauces
Sausages	Tempeh	Infant formulas
Soaps and moisturizers	Processed meats	Low-fat peanut butter
Canned tuna and meat	Canned broths and soups	
High-protein energy bars and snacks	Dairy products (e.g. ice cream, yogurt)	Medications and personal care products

Certain foods and items may not always contain allergens, but soy may show up in unexpected places. Likewise, if you're ever unclear about an item's ingredients, check food labels and feel free to inquire.

Studies reveal that soy allergies typically manifest in early life and are outgrown by the time a child reaches age three. By the time they are ten years old, most kids who have a soy allergy will have overcome it.

Wheat Allergy

1% of children in the United States may be affected by wheat allergy, which is most frequently observed in young children. According to one study, by the time they are 12 years old, two-thirds of youngsters with wheat allergies overcome it. Nonetheless, some people never get over their lifetime allergy to wheat.

A wheat allergy sufferer's immune system produces specialized IgE antibodies that attach to wheat proteins when they are exposed to wheat. Immune system reactions are triggered by this binding and can range in severity from moderate to severe.

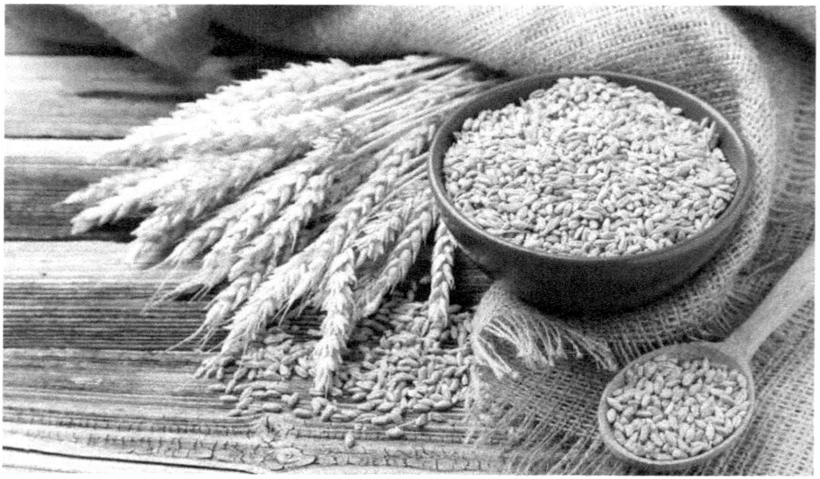

Although they are both unfavorable food reactions, celiac disease and wheat allergy have quite different underlying causes. An unfavorable immune response (IgE-mediated) to wheat proteins causes wheat allergy, which can manifest as classic allergy symptoms in the respiratory system, gastrointestinal tract, skin, and in severe cases, anaphylaxis.

One type of autoimmune illness is celiac disease. Gluten causes the body to create antibodies, which in turn cause inflammation and damage to the lining of the small intestine. The gastrointestinal system is involved in several symptoms (e.g., diarrhea, constipation, weight loss, stomach pain, and bloating). Skin rashes and conditions brought on by dietary deficits are examples of additional symptoms. Similar to wheat allergy, the estimated global prevalence of celiac disease is 1%.

To avoid both immediate and long-term problems, it's critical to collaborate with your doctor in order to get an accurate diagnosis.

Neutralizing Allergic Reaction to Wheat

A wheat allergy reaction can cause modest symptoms like hives or severe symptoms like anaphylaxis. Unpredictably, even very little amounts of wheat might trigger an allergic reaction.

Always carry an epinephrine injection device if you have a wheat allergy. The primary line of treatment for anaphylaxis is epinephrine.

Refraining from Eating Foods That Might Include Wheat (below are a few)

It's crucial that you stay away from wheat and anything that contains wheat to avoid a reaction. Before consuming anything that you haven't cooked yourself, always check the food labels and inquire about the ingredients.

The most widely consumed grain in the US is wheat. All other common grains, with the possible exception of barley, are rarely allergenic to patients with wheat allergy. You still have a large range of meals to choose from, but the grain source needs to be something other than wheat. Search for additional grains including tapioca, amaranth, rye, corn, oats, quinoa, and barley.

The best flour for baking is typically a blend of wheat-free flours. Try out different mixes to determine which one gives you the desired texture.

Within the ingredient list or in a separate "Contains" statement on the packaging, wheat is one of the eight major allergens that federal law requires to be stated in plain language on packaged foods sold in the United States. Because of this, determining whether a food item contains wheat is simple.

Items containing wheat or any of the following ingredients should be avoided:

Bread crumbs	Bulgur	Cereal extract

Club wheat	Couscous	Cracker meal
Durum	Einkorn	Emmer
Farina	Farro	Freekeh
Kamut®	Pasta	Seitan
Semolina	Spelt	Triticale
Sprouted wheat	Vital wheat gluten	Sprouted wheat
Wheat bran hydrolysate	Hydrolyzed wheat protein	Whole wheat berries
Wheat germ oil	Wheat protein isolate	Whole wheat berries
Flour (all-purpose, bread, cake, durum, enriched, graham, high-gluten, high-protein, instant, pastry, self-rising, soft wheat, steel ground, stone ground, whole wheat)	Matzoh, matzo meal (also spelled as matzo, matzah or matzo)	Wheat (bran, durum, germ, gluten, grass, malt, sprouts, starch) Wheat grass

NB: Because it is unrelated to wheat, buckwheat is safe to consume.

The following items occasionally include wheat:

Glucose syrup	Soy sauce	Surimi
Starch (gelatinized starch, modified starch, modified food starch, vegetable starch)	Plant-based meat alternatives	

Numerous Unexpected Wheat Sources

Ale	Baked goods	Baking mixes
Beer	Candy	Crackers
Hot dogs	Breaded foods	Ice cream
Batter-fried foods	Breakfast cereals	Imitation crab meat
Marinara sauce	Processed meats	Salad dressings
Turkey patties	Potato chips	Rice cakes
Sauces	Sausages	Spices
Soups	Play dough or modeling clay	Personal care items (e.g. cosmetics or hair products)
Asian dishes can feature wheat flour flavored	Country-style wreaths are often decorated	

and shaped to look like beef, pork and shrimp.	with wheat products	

These foods and goods don't always contain allergens, although wheat might show up in unexpected places. Read food labels once more, especially if you don't often anticipate seeing wheat. Inquire if you have any questions concerning the ingredients of a product.

Tree Nut Allergy

One of the most prevalent food allergies in both children and adults is tree nut allergy. The six types of tree nuts to which allergies are most frequently reported by both adults and children are cashew, pistachio, walnut, almond, hazelnut, and pecan.

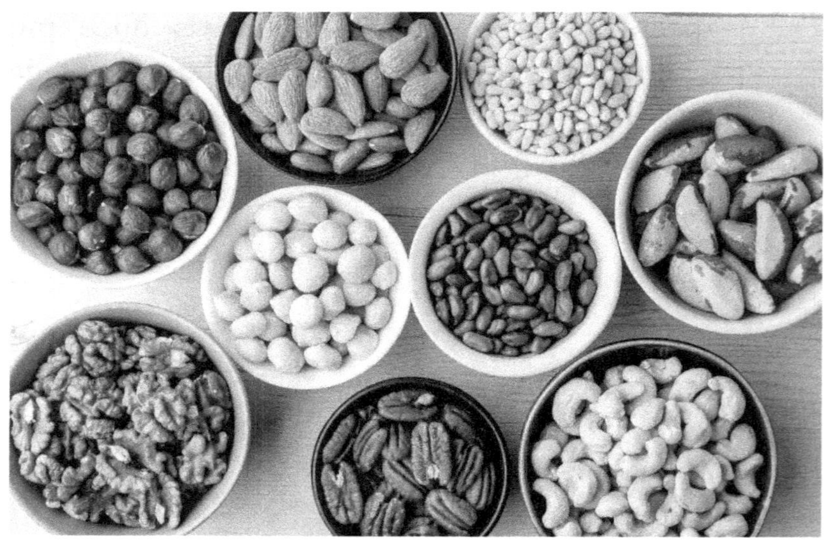

One tree nut allergy affects about 50% of children who also have allergies to other tree nuts. About two thirds of people who have a cashew or walnut sensitivity will also have a pistachio or pecan sensitivity. The majority of kids who have nut allergies do not get over their nut allergy.

Certain IgE antibodies produced by the immune system attach to proteins in nuts when an individual with a nut allergy is exposed to those nuts. Immune system reactions are triggered by this binding and can range in severity from moderate to severe.

Within the United States, 18 distinct types of tree nuts must be labeled on packaged foods using plain language. These tree nuts are not the same as peanuts, which are subterranean legumes related to beans and peas, and only 40% of children with tree nut allergies also have a peanut allergy. Asses, sunflower, poppy, and mustard seeds are seed allergies that do not grow on trees; in contrast, tree nuts do.

Neutralizing Allergic Reaction to Tree nut

Anaphylaxis, a serious allergic reaction that can be fatal, can be brought on by tree nuts. Tree nuts can trigger severe allergic reactions in relatively tiny quantities, and allergic reactions can be erratic.

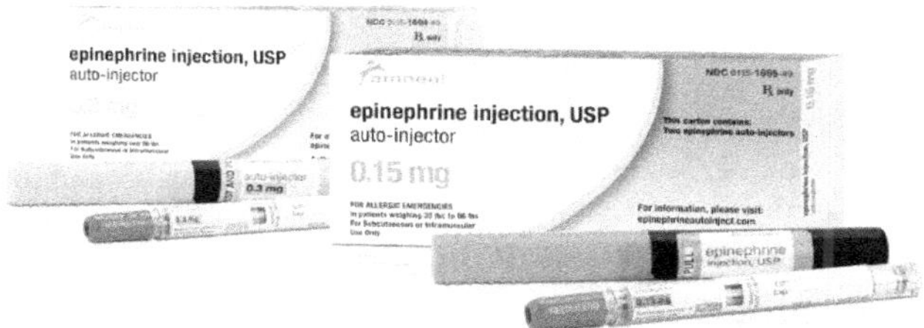

Always carry an epinephrine injection device if you have a tree nut allergy. The primary therapy for anaphylaxis is epinephrine.

Refraining from Eating Foods That Might Include Tree Nut (below are a few)

It's crucial that you stay away from all tree nuts and tree nut-derived items to avoid having a reaction.

You are more likely to be allergic to other varieties of tree nuts if you are allergic to one kind. Your doctor could advise you to stay away from all nuts as a result. It's possible that you'll be told not to eat peanuts due to the increased risk of cross-contamination with tree nuts during production and processing. Your allergist should address and further assess these concerns; perhaps, targeted allergy testing is necessary.

According to federal law, tree nuts are one of the eight main allergens that must be disclosed in plain English on packaged foods sold in the United States. This information must be included in the ingredient list or a separate "Contains" statement on the box. The box for tree nuts has to specify the particular kind. This makes it simple to determine whether a food item contains tree nuts.

Steer clear of anything with tree nuts or any of the following ingredients:

Almond	Artificial nuts	Beechnut
Cashew	Chestnut	Coconut

Chinquapin nut	Filbert/hazelnut	Macadamia nut
Brazil nut	Ginkgo nut	Hickory nut
Nangai nut	Nut meal	Nut meat
Pecan	Pesto	Pili nut
Praline	Walnut	Shea nut
Nut pieces	Pistachio	Marzipan/almond paste
Nut milk (e.g., almond milk, cashew milk)	Nut paste (e.g., almond paste)	Nut oils (e.g., walnut oil, almond oil)
Nut butters (e.g., cashew butter)	Walnut hull extract (flavoring)	Nut distillates/alcoholic extracts
Litchi/lichee/lychee nut	Black walnut hull extract (flavoring)	Gianduja (a chocolate-nut mixture)
Pine nut (also referred to as Indian, pignoli, pignolia, pignon, piñon and pinyon nut)	Natural nut extract (e.g., almond, walnut—although artificial extracts are generally safe)	Butternut (also known as white walnuts; not squash)

Some Unexpected Sources of Tree Nuts

Unexpectedly, flavored coffee, cereals, crackers, biscuits, candies, chocolates, energy bars, frozen desserts, marinades, barbecue sauces, and even cold meats, including mortadella, include tree nut proteins.

For those who have a tree nut allergy, ice cream stores, bakeries, coffee shops, and some restaurants (such as Chinese, African, Indian, Thai, and Vietnamese) are at high risk. The risk of cross-contact is considerable, even if you request a dish that is free of tree nuts.

Lotions, hair care products, and soaps occasionally contain tree nut oils, like walnut and almond.

Because they are so durable, crushed walnut shells can be used to make "natural" sponges or brushes.

It is advisable to steer clear of alcoholic beverages as well, as some of them could include nut flavoring. You might need to contact the producer to find out if natural flavoring and other additives are safe, as these drinks are not subject to federal regulation.

Traditionally, the consumption of coconut, which is the seed of a drupaceous fruit, has not been restricted for those allergic to tree nuts. Nonetheless, the Food and Drug Administration in the United States started classifying coconut as a tree nut in October 2006. Only a tiny number of allergy reactions to coconut have been reported in medical literature; the majority of these events included non-tree nut allergic individuals.

No responses to shea nut oil or butter have been reported, and there is just one example of someone responding to coconut oil that has been documented. A response to one of these would therefore be incredibly unusual.

Seldom have allergic responses to argan oil—which is made from the nut of the argan tree—been documented. In Morocco, you can frequently get this dish, even if it is uncommon in the United States.

Individuals who have a cashew allergy may be more susceptible to developing a pink peppercorn allergy (also known as Brazilian pepper, Rose pepper, Christmasberry, and other names). Different from regular black pepper and fruits with the word "pepper" in their names (such as bell peppers, red peppers, or chili peppers), this dried berry (Schinus, related to cashew) is used as a spice.

NB: Although allergens aren't always present in certain foods and goods, it's still best to be cautious. It is advisable to peruse food labels and inquire about ingredients prior to consuming anything that you have not personally cooked.

Will my child's allergy toTree nuts ever go away?

An allergy to tree nuts tends to be lifelong. Research shows that about 9 percent of children with a tree nut allergy eventually outgrow their allergy.[1]

Younger siblings of children who are allergic to tree nuts may be at higher risk for atopic disease. Every case is different and your doctor can provide guidance about food allergy testing for siblings if appropriate.

Shellfish Allergy

The most prevalent food allergies in adults and among the most prevalent in children are those related to shellfish. An allergy to shellfish is reported by about 2% of Americans.One Allergies to shellfish are often chronic.

The initial allergic reaction occurs in adults for about 60% of those who have a shellfish allergy.

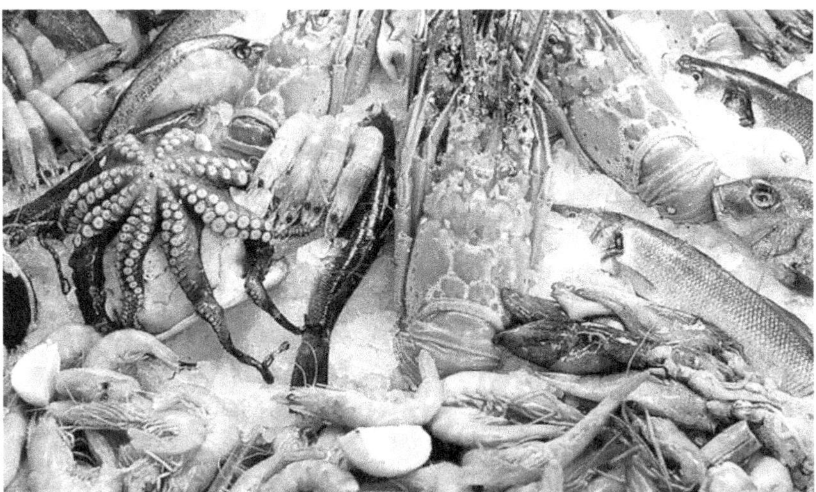

Certain IgE antibodies produced by the immune system of an individual with a shellfish allergy attach to proteins in the shellfish when the individual is exposed to it. The person's immune system is triggered by this, which might result in minor or quite severe reaction symptoms.

Shellfish can be divided into two categories: mollusks/bivalves (which include clams, mussels, oysters, scallops, octopus, squid, abalone, and snail) and crustaceans (which include shrimp, prawns, crab, and lobster). More people have allergies to crustaceans than to mollusks, with shrimp being the most prevalent shellfish allergen in both adults and children.

Shellfish are not closely related to finned fish. If you have an allergy to one, you do not necessarily have to avoid the other, however you should take precautions to keep fish and shellfish from coming into contact. Have a thorough conversation about this matter with your allergist to ensure that the proper dietary restrictions are put in place.

Neutralizing Allergic Reaction to Shellfish

Severe and sometimes fatal allergic responses (including anaphylaxis) can be brought on by shellfish. Even minute amounts of shellfish can trigger an allergic reaction, which can be quite unpredictable.

Have an epinephrine injection kit on you at all times if you are allergic to shellfish. The primary therapy for anaphylaxis is epinephrine.

Refraining from Eating Foods That Might Include Shellfish (below are a few)

Avoiding all shellfish and shellfish products is crucial to preventing a response. Before consuming anything that you haven't cooked yourself, always check the food labels and inquire about the ingredients.

Most persons with shellfish allergies also have allergies to other kinds of shellfish. Generally, your allergist will advise against eating any type of shellfish. If you would want to consume other shellfish but are allergic to a particular kind, discuss with your doctor the possibility of additional allergy testing.

Avoid seafood restaurants as there is a significant chance of cross-contamination between food items. Additionally, you should refrain from traveling to fish markets and handling shellfish. You could be at risk if you're in any area where shellfish are being cooked since the steam may contain protein from the shellfish.

One of the eight main allergens that, according to federal law, must be disclosed in plain English on packaged foods sold in the United States is crustacean shellfish. This information must appear in the ingredient list or a separate "Contains" statement on the packaging. The particular variety, such as crab or shrimp, of crustacean shellfish must also be identified on the packaging. In the United States, mollusks are not currently required to be labeled and may appear in food items without warning.

Avoid foods that contain shellfish or any of these ingredients:

Barnacle	Crab	Krill
Prawns	Shrimp (crevette, scampi)	Crawfish (crawdad, crayfish, ecrevisse)
Lobster (langouste, langoustine, Moreton bay bugs, scampi, tomalley)		

Your doctor may advise you to avoid mollusks* or these ingredients:

Abalone	Cockle	Cuttlefish
Mussels	Octopus	Oysters
Periwinkle	Sea urchin	Scallops
Snails (escargot)	Squid (calamari)	Sea cucumber
Whelk (Turban shell)	Limpet (lapas, opihi)	Clams (cherrystone,

		geoduck, littleneck, pismo, quahog)

Note: The federal government does not require mollusks to be fully disclosed on product labels.

Shellfish are sometimes found in the following:

Bouillabaisse	Cuttlefish ink	Glucosamine
Fish stock	Surimi	
Seafood flavoring (e.g., crab or clam extract)	Fish stock or fish sauce (sometimes made from krill)	

How About Iodine and Carrageenan?

"Irish moss," or carrageenan, is not the same as seafood. Red sea algae is used to thicken, stabilize, and emulsify a variety of dishes, including dairy products. For most people with food allergies, it is safe.

Because shellfish is known to include the element iodine, shellfish allergy and iodine allergy can occasionally be mistaken. However, in those who are allergic to shellfish, iodine does not cause the allergic response. A muscle protein known as tropomyosin is the main allergen found in shellfish and is what triggers an allergic reaction. You do not need to be concerned about iodine or radiocontrast material cross-reactions if you have a shellfish allergy. Radiocontrast material can contain iodine and is utilized in some radiographic medical procedures.

Fish Allergy

At 1% of the US population, one of the most prevalent food allergies is finned fish. The fish to which people most frequently reported adverse reactions in one study were cod, salmon, tuna, and catfish.

The first allergic reaction to fish occurs in about 40% of adult fish allergy sufferers.

When an individual with a fish allergy is exposed to that particular species, certain IgE antibodies produced by the immune system attach to proteins in the fish. This sets off the person's immune system, resulting in a range of reaction symptoms from minor to severe.

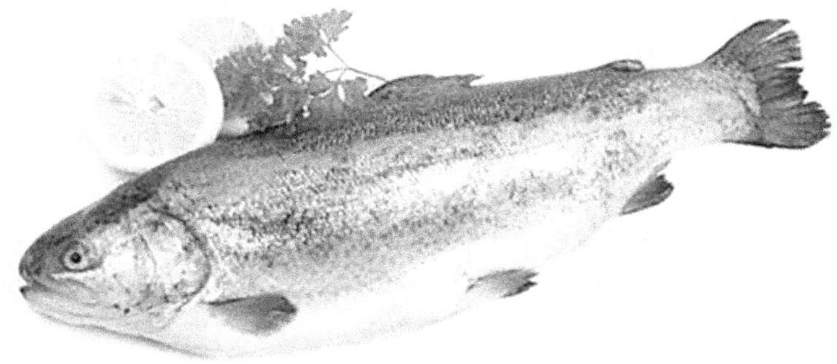

Shellfish are not closely related to finned fish. If you have an allergy to one, you do not necessarily have to avoid the other, however you should take precautions to keep fish and shellfish from coming into contact. Have a thorough conversation about this matter with your allergist to ensure that the proper dietary restrictions are put in place.

Neutralizing Allergic Reaction to Fish

Anaphylaxis and other severe allergic reactions are potentially fatal when triggered by finfish. Unpredictably, even very little amounts of fish might trigger an allergic reaction.

Carry an epinephrine injection kit on you at all times if you are allergic to fish. The primary line of treatment for anaphylaxis is epinephrine.

Refraining from Eating Foods That Might Include Fish (below are a few)

Avoiding all fish and fish products is crucial to preventing a response. Prior to consuming food that you have not personally cooked, always check the labels and inquire about the ingredients.

Food cross-contamination is a major concern in seafood restaurants, so avoid going there. Going to fish markets and handling fish are additional things you should avoid doing. The steam from cooking fish may contain fish protein, therefore you should avoid any location where fish is being prepared.

Most individuals who have a fish allergy also have a fish allergy in over half of cases. You should normally avoid any fish, according to your allergist's advice. If you wish to eat other fish but are allergic to a particular kind, discuss with your doctor about recommended allergy testing.

Listed in plain English either in the ingredient list or in a separate "Contains" statement on the packaging, finfish is one of the eight major allergens that federal law has to be disclosed on packaged goods sold in the United States. Because of this, determining whether a food item contains finned fish is simple.

Fish come in over 20,000 different species. While not an exhaustive list, allergic reactions have frequently been linked to:

Anchovies	Bass	Catfish
Cod	Flounder	Grouper
Haddock	Hake	Halibut
Mahi mahi	Herring	Perch
Pike	Pollock	Salmon
Scrod	Sole	Snapper
Swordfish	Tilapia	Trout

Tuna		

Steer clear of these fish products as well:

Oil Fish Fish Flavoring	Fish gelatin, made from the skin and bones of fish	Fish sticks (some people make the mistake of thinking these don't contain real fish)

Numerous Unexpected Fish Sources

Barbecue sauce	Bouillabaisse	Caesar salad and Caesar dressing
Caponata, a Sicilian eggplant relish	Imitation or artificial fish or shellfish (e.g., surimi, also known as "sea legs" or "sea sticks")	Worcestershire sauce

While fish can turn up in unexpected places, allergens aren't always present in these foods and goods. Once more, if you're ever unclear about an item's ingredients, read food labels and ask questions.

Sesame Allergy

In the United States, sesame allergies rank tenth among food allergies in both children and adults. In the US, 0.23 percent of adults and children have a sesame allergy. From baked products to sushi, the edible seeds of the sesame plant are a ubiquitous element in cuisines throughout. Over the past 20 years, there have been several reports suggesting a considerable global increase in cases of this allergy.

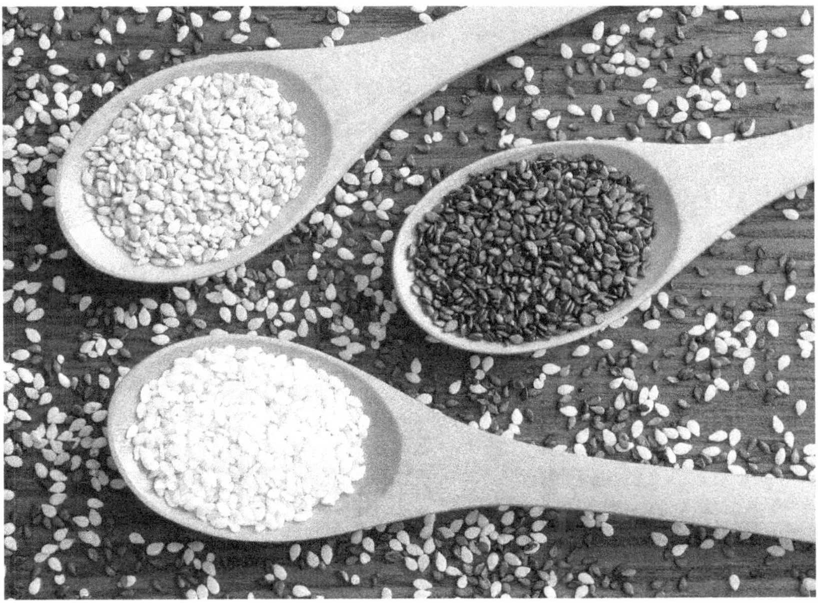

Certain IgE antibodies produced by the immune system of an individual with a sesame allergy attach to proteins in the sesame when the individual is exposed to sesame. Reaction symptoms might range from minor to severe as a result of the person's immune system being triggered.

Sesame was required to be listed as a major allergy on packaged foods in the United States as of January 1, 2023, and its labels must be in plain language. Until new inventory is added, products made before 2023 might still include unmarked sesame, which will stay on store shelves.

Neutralizing Allergic Reaction to Sesame

Each person has a different level of sensitivity to sesame, and reactions can be unexpected. Sesame allergy reactions can cause modest symptoms like hives or severe symptoms like anaphylaxis.

If you are allergic to sesame, carry an epidural needle with you at all times. The primary line of treatment for anaphylaxis is epinephrine.

Refraining from Eating Foods That Might Include Sesame (below are a few)

It's critical to stay away from sesame in order to stop a reaction. Numerous unusual names can be used for the same substances.

Before consuming anything that you have not personally cooked, always check the labels on food products and inquire about the components.

Steer clear of anything with sesame or any of the following ingredients:

Sesame flour	Sesame oil	Sesame paste
Sesame salt	Sesame seed	Sesamol
Halvah	Semolina	Sim sim
Sesamum indicum	Tahini, Tahina, Tehina	Til
Benne, benne seed, benniseed	Gingelly, gingelly oil	Gomasio (sesame salt)

Research indicates that the majority of individuals with particular food protein allergies can consume highly refined oils derived from such foods without any problems (very refined peanut and soybean oil are two examples). Those who are allergic to sesame should stay away from sesame oil because it is not highly refined.

Sesame in Spices or Flavorings

Sesame may be included without being declared in components like flavors or spice mixes in packaged foods produced before January 1, 2023. Inquire about the manufacturer's ingredients and manufacturing procedures over the phone if you are unclear if a product may contain sesame.

Flavoring recipes and spice blends are regarded as confidential knowledge. It is possible that the manufacturer is unable to provide the whole list of ingredients. Ask whether sesame is used as an ingredient specifically instead.

Foods That May Contain Sesame

Soups	Sushi	Tempeh
Vegetarian burgers	Turkish cake	Falafel
Margarine	Hummus	Bread crumbs
Pasteli (Greek dessert)	Processed meats and sausages	Protein and energy bars
Dressings, gravies, marinades and sauces	Goma-dofu (Japanese dessert)	Herbs and herbal drinks
Chips (such as bagel chips, pita chips and tortilla chips)	Crackers (such as melba toast and sesame snap bars)	Cereals (such as granola and muesli)

Asian cuisine (sesame oil is commonly used in cooking)	Baked goods (such as bagels, bread, breadsticks, hamburger buns and rolls)	Dipping sauces (such as baba ganoush, hummus and tahini sauce)
Flavored rice, noodles, risotto, shish kebabs, stews and stir fry	Snack foods (such as pretzels, candy, Halvah, Japanese snack mix and rice cakes)	

These foods and goods don't necessarily contain allergens, but sesame might turn up in unexpected places. Once more, if you have any queries concerning an item's ingredients, study the food labels.

In conclusion, the best treatment, control, and prevention method for combating and putting a stop to the afflictions imposed on us by these allergic foods is **abstinence**. And always remember that "your health is your wealth," so be serious about abiding by the abstinence rules of the above-listed foods if any are your allergy trigger sources. No more gambling with our health.